LIP BALM FOR BEGINNERS

Essential Guide To Homemade Chapstick
Recipes, Ingredients, Techniques, Tips For
Healthy, Nourishing And Hydrating Your Lips

ALFORD BARTELL

DISCLAIMER

The author of this book is not linked, associated, authorized, sponsored, or otherwise related to any corporation, business, or person mentioned in this book. This book was written based on the author's expertise, insight, and personal experiences. The material given is intended for educational and informative purposes only and should not be construed as professional advice. The author and publisher accept no responsibility or liability for any mistakes or omissions in the contents of this book. All thoughts stated are solely those of the author and do not represent the views of any organizations.

Table of Contents

ABOUT THIS BOOK

This book "Lip Balm" serves as an essential guide for anyone interested in the art and science of crafting their lip care products. It meticulously explores the advantages of homemade lip balm, emphasizing how it can be a healthier, more personalized alternative to commercial products. The introduction covers not only the benefits of creating your lip balm but also provides an overview of essential ingredients and the necessary tools and equipment. This foundation ensures readers understand both the practical and safety aspects of lip balm making, from basic safety precautions to the nuances of different lip balm bases.

A significant portion of this book is dedicated to detailing the selection of essential ingredients. It offers guidance on choosing the right oils, understanding the role of beeswax and its alternatives, and incorporating natural butter and essential oils. This section highlights how these components contribute to the moisturizing and therapeutic properties of the balm, as well as the potential for adding natural colorants and additives to enhance the product.

Tools and equipment are thoroughly addressed, with a focus on the essential tools needed for lip balm production. This book provides insight into different types of containers, safety gear, and where to source equipment. This information equips readers with the knowledge to set up their workspace efficiently and safely.

The step-by-step guide to making basic lip balm walks readers through the entire process, from preparing the workspace and melting ingredients to pouring the mixture into containers and cooling the final product.

This practical approach ensures that even beginners can create high-quality lip balm with ease.

Customization is a key feature of the book, offering detailed instructions on how to adjust the firmness and consistency of the balm, create tinted variations, add SPF protection, and experiment with flavors. It also addresses the needs of those who prefer vegan or allergen-free alternatives, showcasing the flexibility and creativity involved in lip balm formulation.

Common issues encountered in lip balm making are addressed with troubleshooting tips, providing solutions for problems such as hardness, graininess, and separation. This section helps readers overcome challenges and refine their techniques.

Packaging and labeling are explored with a focus on eco-friendly options, attractive designs, and compliance with labeling regulations. This guidance supports readers in presenting their products professionally and appealingly, enhancing their marketability.

This book also covers essential storage and shelf life guidelines, advising on the best practices for keeping homemade lip balm fresh and extending its usability. It provides tips for testing freshness and knowing when to discard old batches.

Finally, this book delves into the enjoyment and benefits of using homemade lip balm, offering insights into incorporating it into daily routines and sharing creations with others. It includes feedback from experienced users and tips for those interested in exploring advanced techniques, such as creating specialty lip balms or starting a small business.

CHAPTER ONE

Introduction To Making Your Lip Balm

Understanding The Benefits Of Homemade Lip Balm

Creating your lip balm at home offers numerous benefits that store-bought options might not provide. Homemade lip balm allows you to control the ingredients and tailor the formulation to meet your specific needs, which is especially advantageous if you have sensitive skin or allergies. By making lip balm yourself, you avoid synthetic chemicals and preservatives commonly found in commercial products, opting instead for natural, nourishing ingredients that can be more beneficial for your lips.

Another advantage is the customization aspect. You can choose from a wide range of essential oils and natural flavors to create a lip balm that suits your personal preferences. This customization not only enhances the sensory experience of using the lip balm but also allows you to experiment with different formulations, such as adding SPF for sun protection or incorporating antioxidants for extra skin benefits. Homemade lip balm also makes for thoughtful, personalized gifts, as you can create unique blends that reflect the recipient's tastes.

Making your lip balm can also be more cost-effective than buying high-end products. With basic ingredients and a few essential tools, you can produce multiple batches of lip balm for a fraction of the price of store-bought versions. This aspect of DIY lip balm appeals to those looking to save money while enjoying a high-quality, personalized product.

To make your lip balm, you'll need a few essential ingredients that form the foundation of a good formulation. These typically include a base (such as beeswax or shea butter), oils for moisturizing (like coconut oil or sweet almond oil), and optional additives like flavorings or colorants.

1. Beeswax: This is a key ingredient that helps to solidify the lip balm and provide a protective barrier for your lips. Beeswax also has natural antibacterial properties, which can help prevent infections and keep your lips healthy.

2. Carrier Oils: These oils, such as coconut oil, sweet almond oil, or jojoba oil, are crucial for moisturizing and nourishing your lips. They add softness and hydration, ensuring that your lip balm isn't just protective but also soothing and emollient.

3. Butter: Ingredients like shea butter or cocoa butter can be added for their rich, creamy texture and additional moisturizing properties. They help to make the lip balm more luxurious and effective at softening and conditioning your lips.

4. Flavorings and Colorants (optional): Natural flavorings, such as peppermint or vanilla extract, and colorants can be added to give your lip balm a pleasant scent and a touch of color. Ensure that any additives are lip-safe and free from harmful chemicals.

Tools And Equipment Needed

Making lip balm at home requires a few basic tools and equipment to ensure that the process goes smoothly. Here's a list of what you'll need:

1. Double Boiler or Heatproof Bowl: A double boiler is ideal for gently melting the beeswax and oils without burning them. If you don't have one, you can use a heatproof bowl placed over a pot of simmering water.

2. Stirring Utensils: Wooden spoons or spatulas are used to mix the ingredients. Avoid using metal utensils if you are working with essential oils, as they can react with the metal.

3. Lip Balm Containers: You'll need small containers or tubes to hold your finished lip balm. These can be purchased online or repurposed from old lip balm containers.

4. Measuring Tools: Accurate measurement is crucial for consistency. Use measuring spoons and cups to ensure that you get the right proportions of each ingredient.

5. Pipettes or Droppers (optional): For precise addition of flavorings and colorants, pipettes or

droppers can be helpful. They allow you to add small amounts without overdoing it.

6. Labels: If you plan to gift or sell your lip balm, consider labeling your containers with the ingredients and date of production.

Basic Safety Precautions

When making lip balm, it's important to follow some basic safety precautions to ensure that your product is both safe and effective.

1. Hygiene: Always start with clean hands and work surfaces. Clean all equipment thoroughly before use to avoid contamination. This prevents any potential bacteria or mold from entering your lip balm mixture.

2. Temperature Control: When melting beeswax and oils, do so at a low temperature to avoid overheating. High temperatures can degrade the quality of your ingredients and result in a poor texture.

3. Allergies: Conduct a patch test with any new ingredient to ensure that you do not have an allergic reaction. This is particularly important for essential oils and flavorings, which can sometimes irritate.

4. Storage: Store your lip balm in a cool, dry place to prolong its shelf life. Avoid exposing it to direct sunlight or heat, which can cause the product to melt or degrade.

Introduction To Different Lip Balm Bases

Lip balm bases serve as the foundation for your homemade product. Understanding the different types can help you choose the right one for your needs.

1. Beeswax Base: Beeswax is a popular choice for creating a solid, durable lip balm. It provides a protective layer on the lips and is known for its natural, soothing properties. Beeswax bases are ideal for those who prefer a traditional, well-established formula.

2. Shea Butter Base: Shea butter offers a rich, creamy texture that melts smoothly on the lips. It is highly moisturizing and ideal for those with dry or sensitive lips. Shea butter bases are often used in more luxurious, hydrating lip balms.

3. Coconut Oil Base: Coconut oil is known for its moisturizing and antimicrobial properties. It creates a soft, smooth lip balm that is excellent for daily use. Coconut oil bases can be blended with other oils and butter for added benefits.

4. Vegan Bases: For those who prefer a vegan option, there are plant-based alternatives to

beeswax, such as candelilla wax or carnauba wax. These vegan bases can be used to create a lip balm that is both effective and cruelty-free.

By understanding these basics, you can confidently start making your lip balm at home, ensuring a personalized and satisfying experience.

CHAPTER TWO

Essential Ingredients For Homemade Lip Balm

Choosing The Right Oils For Your Lip Balm

When making homemade lip balm, selecting the right oils is crucial for achieving the desired texture and moisturizing properties. Start by understanding the properties of various oils to choose the best combination for your needs. Coconut oil is a popular choice due to its excellent moisturizing and anti-bacterial qualities. It helps create a smooth texture and adds a pleasant scent. Sweet almond oil is another great option, known for its lightweight nature and high vitamin E content, which helps nourish and repair the skin.

Jojoba oil closely resembles the skin's natural oils, making it a fantastic choice for balancing and hydrating lips without feeling greasy. Olive oil is another beneficial option, rich in antioxidants and vitamins, which help to soften and protect your lips. When formulating your lip balm, you might blend these oils to achieve a balanced consistency and maximum moisturizing effect. To ensure optimal results, experiment with different ratios until you find the perfect combination for your skin's needs.

Importance Of Beeswax And Its Alternatives

Beeswax plays a crucial role in homemade lip balm by providing a solid structure and a protective barrier on the lips. It has natural emollient properties that help seal in moisture and prevent your lips from drying out. Beeswax also adds a glossy finish to the lip balm, which can enhance its appeal. To use beeswax, melt it gently using a double boiler, and mix it with your chosen oils until fully incorporated.

For those who prefer vegan options, there are several beeswax alternatives available. Candelilla wax is a popular substitute, derived from the leaves of the candelilla plant. It provides similar benefits to beeswax, including a firm texture and moisture-sealing properties. Carnauba wax is another option, known for its high melting point, which can give your lip balm a firmer texture. Simply substitute these waxes in equal amounts for beeswax in your recipe and follow the same melting and mixing process.

Adding Natural Butter For Moisture

Natural butter is essential for adding richness and moisture to your lip balm. Shea butter is a top choice due to its high content of fatty acids

27

and vitamins, which deeply nourish and hydrate the lips. It also has anti-inflammatory properties that can soothe and repair chapped lips. Cocoa butter is another excellent option, providing a creamy texture and a pleasant scent, while also offering moisturizing benefits.

To incorporate butter into your lip balm, gently melt it along with your oils and wax using a double boiler. Once melted, mix thoroughly to ensure an even distribution of the butter throughout the balm. Adjust the amount of butter based on your preferred texture; more butter will create a richer, thicker balm, while less will result in a lighter, smoother product. Experiment with different kinds of butter or combinations to find the ideal formula for your lip balm.

Essential oils not only add a delightful fragrance to your homemade lip balm but also provide therapeutic benefits. For instance, peppermint oil gives a refreshing, tingly sensation and can help soothe dry, cracked lips. Lavender oil is known for its calming properties and can promote healing. Tea tree oil has antiseptic properties that are beneficial for protecting lips from infections.

When adding essential oils to your lip balm, start with a small amount and gradually increase based on your preference. Typically, 5-10 drops per batch is sufficient. Be cautious with strong essential oils, as they can be irritating if used in excess. Mix the essential oils into your melted lip balm mixture before pouring them into containers, ensuring they are evenly distributed for consistent fragrance and benefits.

Incorporating Natural Colorants And Additives

Adding natural colorants and additives can enhance the visual appeal and effectiveness of your homemade lip balm. Beetroot powder is a natural option for adding a reddish tint, while cocoa powder can provide a subtle brown shade. For a touch of shimmer, consider adding a small amount of mica powder.

When incorporating colorants, start with a small amount and mix thoroughly to achieve the desired shade. Add these ingredients to your melted mixture before pouring it into containers. For exfoliating benefits, you can also add finely ground sugar or coffee grounds. These additives should be mixed into the balm right before pouring it into containers to ensure an even distribution.

By following these guidelines and experimenting with different ingredients, you can create a variety of personalized lip balms that cater to your specific needs and preferences.

CHAPTER THREE

Tools And Equipment Needed

Essential Tools For Lip Balm Making

To start making your lip balm, you'll need a few essential tools. These tools ensure that the process is efficient, safe, and enjoyable. Here's a list of what you'll need:

1. **Double Boiler or Heatproof Bowl and Pot:** A double boiler is ideal for melting waxes and butter, as it provides gentle, even heat. If you don't have a double boiler, you can use a heatproof bowl set over a pot of simmering water. This setup prevents direct heat from scorching your ingredients.

2. **Measuring Spoons and Cups:** Accurate measurements are crucial in lip balm making.

Invest in a set of measuring spoons and cups to ensure precise quantities of each ingredient. This accuracy is key to achieving the right consistency and effectiveness of your balm.

3. **Stirring Utensils:** Silicone spatulas or wooden spoons work best for mixing your ingredients. They are durable, heat-resistant, and won't react with your products. A whisk can also be useful if you're incorporating a lot of ingredients.

4. **Thermometer:** A candy or kitchen thermometer will help you monitor the temperature of your melted mixture. This is important to ensure that the balm sets correctly and maintains its intended texture.

5. **Pipettes or Droppers:** If you're adding essential oils or other liquid ingredients, pipettes or droppers provide precision. They help you

control the exact amount of each additive, preventing overuse.

Understanding Different Types Of Containers

Selecting the right container for your lip balm is crucial, not only for functionality but also for presentation. Here are some popular options:

1.   Lip Balm Tubes: These are the most common and convenient containers for lip balm. They come in various sizes and typically have a twist-up mechanism that pushes the balm out. They are portable and easy to apply, making them a favorite choice.

2.   Lip Balm Pots or Jars: Pots offer a more traditional approach, where you use your finger or a small spatula to apply the balm. They are great for home use and allow you to use different formulations or even create custom blends.

3.   **Lip Balm Tins:** Small, round tins are another popular option. They provide a vintage look and can be reused or recycled. Tins are sturdy and protect your balm from external elements, but they require a bit more care during application to avoid contamination.

4.   **Roll-On Containers:** These are less common for homemade lip balms but can be used for liquid or gel-based balms. They offer a smooth application and are good for on-the-go use.

Safety Gear And Precautions

Making lip balm involves handling hot waxes and oils, so safety is paramount. Follow these precautions to ensure a safe experience:

1.   **Wear Heat-Resistant Gloves:** Protect your hands from burns by wearing heat-resistant

gloves, especially when handling hot containers or melting ingredients.

2.   Use Safety Goggles: Safety goggles can protect your eyes from any splashes or accidental spills, particularly when working with hot oils and waxes.

3.   Work in a Clean Area: Ensure your workspace is clean and organized. This minimizes the risk of contamination and makes the process smoother. Wipe down surfaces and use clean utensils for each step.

4.   Avoid Inhalation: Some ingredients may release fumes when heated. Work in a well-ventilated area or use a fan to disperse any vapors. Avoid inhaling fumes directly.

Finding the right equipment is crucial for successful lip balm making. Here are some reliable sources:

1.   **Craft Supply Stores:** These stores often carry a range of tools and containers for DIY projects, including lip balm making. They are a great starting point for beginners looking for specialized equipment.

2.   **Online Retailers:** Websites like Amazon or specialty sites like Bramble Berry offer a wide selection of lip balm-making supplies. You can find everything from measuring tools to containers and ingredients, often with customer reviews to guide your choices.

3.   **Kitchen Supply Stores:** For basic equipment like double boilers, measuring spoons, and

spatulas, kitchen supply stores are a great option. They offer durable tools that are also used in everyday cooking.

4.   Health Food Stores: If you're looking for organic or specialty ingredients, health food stores can be a valuable resource. They often stock essential oils, natural butter, and waxes that are ideal for homemade lip balms.

By gathering these essential tools and understanding how to use them, you'll be well on your way to creating your lip balms. Each piece of equipment plays a vital role in ensuring the final product is both effective and enjoyable to use.

CHAPTER FOUR

Step-By-Step Guide To Making Basic Lip Balm

Preparing Your Workspace

Creating your lip balm starts with setting up a clean, organized workspace. This ensures that all your ingredients remain uncontaminated and the process runs smoothly. Begin by gathering all the necessary supplies: a double boiler or microwave-safe bowl, stirring utensils (like a spatula or spoon), lip balm containers or tubes, and measuring tools. Clean all your equipment thoroughly to avoid introducing any bacteria or impurities into your lip balm mixture.

It's also important to lay down some protective coverings for your work surface to catch any spills or drips.

You can use paper towels or a disposable tablecloth for this purpose. Make sure your workspace is in a well-ventilated area, especially if you're using any essential oils or fragrances that might have strong scents. By preparing your workspace meticulously, you'll minimize the risk of errors and create a pleasant environment for making your lip balm.

Melting And Mixing Ingredients

The next step in making lip balm is melting and mixing the ingredients. Start by measuring out your base ingredients, which typically include beeswax, shea butter, and coconut oil. Beeswax acts as a thickener and provides a solid structure, while shea butter and coconut oil offer moisturizing properties. Place these ingredients into a double boiler or a microwave-safe bowl.

If using a double boiler, heat the mixture over simmering water until it melts completely, stirring occasionally to combine the ingredients evenly. If using a microwave, heat in short intervals of 20-30 seconds, stirring in between, until fully melted. Be cautious not to overheat, as this can degrade the quality of the ingredients. Once the mixture is melted and homogeneous, remove it from heat. If desired, you can also mix in any additional oils or butter at this stage to enhance the balm's properties.

Adding Fragrance And Color

With your base mixture melted and well-combined, it's time to add fragrance and color to personalize your lip balm. Essential oils or flavor oils are commonly used to provide a pleasant scent and taste. For a basic lip balm, start with a few drops of essential oil or flavoring, and mix thoroughly.

Peppermint, lavender, and vanilla are popular choices, but you can experiment with various scents according to your preference.

For coloring, you can use a small amount of lip-safe colorant or even natural ingredients like beetroot powder for a hint of color. Add the colorant to your melted base and stir well to ensure even distribution. Keep in mind that the color may appear more intense in the melted state but will lighten up once the lip balm cools and solidifies. Test the fragrance and color intensity by placing a small amount of the mixture on a spoon and letting it cool to see how it looks and smells.

Pouring Into Containers

Once your lip balm mixture is fully combined and ready, carefully pour it into the containers you have prepared.

If you're using lip balm tubes, ensure they are upright and secure on a tray or plate to prevent spills. If you're using small jars or tins, use a small funnel or dropper to avoid making a mess. Pour the mixture slowly to avoid bubbles and splashes.

Allow the mixture to settle and fill the containers to the desired level. It's a good idea to keep a few extra containers on hand in case you have leftover balm. If the mixture begins to harden before you've finished pouring, gently reheat it until it reaches a liquid state again. Be precise during this step to ensure that each container is filled evenly and that the lip balm maintains a consistent texture and quality.

Cooling And Storing Your Lip Balm

After pouring your lip balm into containers, let it cool and solidify at room temperature. This process can take a few hours, depending on the size of the containers and the ambient temperature. Avoid moving or disturbing the containers during this time to ensure that the lip balm sets evenly without any imperfections.

Once fully cooled and solidified, your lip balm is ready for use. Store the finished lip balms in a cool, dry place away from direct sunlight and heat to maintain their quality. Proper storage helps extend the shelf life of your homemade lip balm and ensures it remains effective and enjoyable to use. If you're gifting the lip balm, consider adding labels or packaging to personalize and protect your creations.

CHAPTER FIVE

Customizing Your Lip Balm Recipes

Adjusting The Firmness And Consistency

To customize the firmness and consistency of your lip balm, you'll need to adjust the ratio of waxes, butter, and oils used in your recipe. The primary ingredients that affect firmness are beeswax (or its alternatives), cocoa butter, and shea butter. Beeswax is the most common choice for adding firmness, while cocoa and shea butter help to soften and moisturize.

Basic Method for Adjusting Firmness:

Determine the Base Ratio: Start with a basic ratio of 2 parts wax, 1 part butter, and 1 part oil. For example, if you use 2 tablespoons of beeswax, add 1 tablespoon each of cocoa butter and a carrier oil like almond oil.

Test the Firmness: Melt the waxes and butter together in a double boiler, then stir in the oils. Pour a small amount into a spoon and let it cool. Test the consistency. If it's too soft, increase the beeswax; if it's too hard, add more oil.

Adjust Gradually: Make adjustments in small increments. For a firmer balm, increase the amount of beeswax or reduce the oil. For a softer balm, add more oil or butter. Keep track of your changes so you can replicate or adjust the formula as needed.

This approach allows you to fine-tune the texture of your lip balm, ensuring it has the perfect consistency for your preference.

Creating tinted lip balms is a fun way to add a splash of color to your products. Tints can be achieved using natural colorants like beet powder, mica powders, or even lipstick.

Basic Method for Adding Tint:

Choose Your Colorant: Select a natural colorant. Beet powder provides a reddish tint, while mica powders come in various shades. Lipstick can be melted into the mixture for a more intense color.

Add Color to the Base: Melt your base of beeswax, butter, and oils. Once melted, add a small amount of your chosen colorant. For powders, start with a pinch and mix thoroughly. For lipstick, chop and melt it into the base.

Test and Adjust: Pour a small amount of the mixture into a spoon and let it cool to test the color. Adjust by adding more colorant if needed. Keep in mind that the color will slightly change as it cools and solidifies.

Experiment with different colorants and combinations to create a range of tinted lip balms, perfect for various moods and occasions.

Adding SPF Protection

Adding SPF (sun protection factor) to your lip balm is a great way to protect your lips from harmful UV rays. Zinc oxide is the most common and effective ingredient for this purpose.

Basic Method for Incorporating SPF:

Select SPF Ingredients: Use non-nano zinc oxide, which is safe for skin application. A general recommendation is to use about 5% zinc oxide in your lip balm for SPF 15 protection.

Blend with the Base: Melt your beeswax, butter, and oils together. Once melted, add the zinc oxide powder and mix thoroughly. Ensure the zinc oxide is evenly distributed to avoid clumping.

Test and Adjust: Pour a small amount of the mixture into a spoon and let it cool. Check the consistency and SPF effectiveness. Adjust the amount of zinc oxide if needed, following safety guidelines for SPF concentrations.

Adding SPF helps protect your lips from sun damage while keeping them moisturized and smooth.

Experimenting With Different Flavors

Experimenting with flavors can enhance the sensory experience of your lip balm. Essential oils and flavor oils are commonly used for this purpose.

Choose Your Flavors: Select food-grade essential oils or flavor oils. Peppermint, vanilla, and citrus are popular choices. Start with a few drops, as essential oils are potent.

Blend with the Base: After melting your base, remove it from heat and stir in the flavor oils. For essential oils, add 2-3 drops per ounce of base. For flavor oils, follow the manufacturer's recommendations.

Test and Adjust: Pour a small amount of the mixture into a spoon and let it cool to test the flavor. Adjust by adding more flavoring if desired.

Experimenting with flavors allows you to create a variety of lip balms that cater to different preferences and enhance the overall user experience.

Creating vegan or allergen-free lip balms involves substituting animal-derived ingredients and ensuring the formula is free of common allergens.

Basic Method for Vegan Lip Balm:

Substitute Waxes: Replace beeswax with plant-based alternatives like candelilla wax or carnauba wax. These provide similar firmness without animal products.

Use Vegan Butters and Oils: Cocoa butter and shea butter are naturally vegan. Ensure all other oils and ingredients are plant-based and allergen-free.

Mix and Test: Melt the vegan waxes and butter together, then add your oils. Follow the same process as traditional lip balm making, adjusting the firmness as needed.

Identify Common Allergens: Avoid ingredients like nuts or soy if making allergen-free balms. Opt for hypoallergenic oils such as jojoba or sunflower oil.

Use Non-Allergenic Ingredients: Choose butter and waxes that are unlikely to cause allergic reactions. Verify that all ingredients are free from common allergens.

Mix and Test: Prepare the balm as usual, ensuring all ingredients are blended well. Conduct a patch test on a small area of skin to confirm there are no adverse reactions.

CHAPTER SIX

Troubleshooting Common Issues

Lip Balm Too Hard Or Too Soft

When crafting your lip balm, achieving the perfect consistency is crucial. If your lip balm turns out too hard, it can be uncomfortable to apply, while a balm that is too soft may not provide the desired protection or could be prone to melting. To troubleshoot this issue, start by understanding the ratios and properties of the ingredients you use.

Hard Lip Balm

A lip balm that is too hard usually has too much solid fat or wax compared to the oils. To fix this, you need to adjust the balance of your ingredients.

For instance, if you use too much beeswax, which is a common cause of hardness, reduce the amount in your next batch. Beeswax creates a firm consistency, so reducing it slightly and increasing the amount of carrier oils, like coconut oil or shea butter, can soften the balm. You can also try adding a small amount of lanolin or cocoa butter, which will help to balance the texture.

Soft Lip Balm

Conversely, if your lip balm is too soft, you have likely used too much oil or not enough wax. To correct this, increase the proportion of beeswax or another solid fat in your recipe. This will help to thicken the balm and give it a more solid consistency. Make sure to melt and blend the ingredients thoroughly to achieve a uniform texture.

If you've already made the balm, you can reheat it, adjust the proportions, and pour it back into the containers.

Dealing With Grainy Textures

A grainy texture in lip balm usually results from the crystallization of ingredients or improper mixing. This can be bothersome as it affects the smoothness of the application.

Causes and Solutions

Graininess often occurs when butter, such as shea butter or cocoa butter, is not fully melted before mixing. To prevent this, ensure that all your solid ingredients are completely melted before combining them with oils. Use a double boiler for gentle and even heating, which helps to avoid overheating and thus crystallization. Stir the mixture thoroughly to ensure a smooth blend.

If your lip balm has already cooled and developed a grainy texture, you can melt it down again, ensuring it stirs well while it's in the liquid state. Once melted, allow it to cool slowly to help prevent the formation of crystals. Also, adding a small amount of a stabilizer, such as a silicone-based ingredient, can help in achieving a smoother texture.

Lip Balm Not Setting Properly

If your lip balm is not set properly, it might be due to an incorrect balance of ingredients or cooling issues. Proper setting ensures that the balm maintains its shape and texture.

Solutions

Ensure that your recipe has the correct ratio of wax to oils. Too little wax will prevent the balm from solidifying properly.

If you find your lip balm isn't setting as expected, you can increase the amount of beeswax or another solid fat. Reheat the mixture, add a bit more wax, and stir well before pouring it into containers.

Cooling is also an essential factor. Lip balm should be cooled slowly and at room temperature to set properly. Avoid placing it in the refrigerator as rapid cooling can lead to separation or other texture issues. Let it cool undisturbed to allow it to set correctly.

Addressing Separation Issues

Separation in lip balm happens when the oil and wax components don't stay uniformly mixed, leading to an uneven texture.

Prevention and Fixes

To prevent separation, make sure that all ingredients are thoroughly mixed while they are still in a liquid state. This can be achieved by continuously stirring the mixture during cooling to ensure an even distribution of the ingredients.

If separation has already occurred, you can reheat the balm to re-melt the mixture, then stir it well before allowing it to cool again. Ensure that the container used is clean and free from moisture, as this can contribute to separation.

Preventing Mold And Bacteria Growth

Ensuring your lip balm is free from mold and bacteria is essential for safety and effectiveness. Proper hygiene and ingredient handling plays a significant role in this.

Hygiene Practices

Use clean tools and containers when preparing and storing your lip balm. Any contamination from utensils or containers can introduce bacteria or mold spores. Sterilize containers and tools before use, and ensure your working area is clean.

Additionally, consider adding natural preservatives like Vitamin E oil, which has antimicrobial properties and helps extend the shelf life of your lip balm. Store the finished lip balm in a cool, dry place away from direct sunlight, and always check for any signs of spoilage before use. If you notice any changes in color, texture, or smell, it's best to discard the product and make a fresh batch.

CHAPTER SEVEN

Packaging And Labeling Your Lip Balm

Choosing Eco-Friendly Packaging Options

When it comes to packaging your lip balm, opting for eco-friendly options not only aligns with sustainable practices but also appeals to environmentally-conscious consumers. Start by exploring materials such as biodegradable or recyclable containers. Glass jars and aluminum tins are excellent choices for those looking to avoid plastic. These materials can be recycled or reused, reducing waste and environmental impact.

For a more innovative approach, consider using compostable packaging made from plant-based materials like cornstarch or sugarcane.

These options break down naturally in composting environments, leaving a minimal environmental footprint. If you prefer a more conventional route, look for suppliers who offer post-consumer recycled plastic, which utilizes plastic that has already been recycled once, helping to close the recycling loop.

In addition to selecting sustainable materials, think about the size and design of your packaging. Smaller, compact containers often use fewer materials, which contributes to overall sustainability. Ensure that your packaging is functional and practical for users, making it easy to apply the lip balm without unnecessary waste.

Designing Attractive Labels

Designing an attractive label is crucial for grabbing the attention of potential customers and conveying your brand's identity.

Start by selecting a design that reflects the essence of your lip balm. This could include using colors, fonts, and images that align with the fragrance or benefits of the product. For example, a lip balm with a soothing lavender scent might feature calming purple tones and images of lavender flowers.

Incorporate high-quality graphics and professional design elements to ensure your label stands out on the shelf. Utilize graphic design software or hire a designer if needed, to create a label that is visually appealing and well-organized. Your design should also include practical elements, such as clear and legible text for product details.

Ensure that your labels are durable and resistant to moisture, as lip balm is often used in various environments. Waterproof or laminated labels are ideal for this purpose.

Additionally, consider incorporating features like a tamper-evident seal to enhance product safety and integrity.

Including Necessary Product Information

Accurate and comprehensive product information is essential for informing your customers and meeting regulatory requirements. Your label should include the product name, a list of ingredients, and any relevant warnings or usage instructions. For lip balm, highlighting key ingredients such as natural oils or organic components can attract health-conscious consumers.

Provide clear directions on how to use the product and any specific storage instructions to ensure optimal performance and longevity. For example, indicate if the lip balm should be stored in a cool, dry place to maintain its consistency. Additionally, include your contact information or website for customer inquiries and feedback.

To comply with labeling regulations, make sure to include any required disclaimers or certifications. This could include allergy information, certifications like cruelty-free or vegan, or adherence to specific cosmetic regulations. Check local and international guidelines to ensure your labeling meets all necessary legal standards.

Compliance With Labeling Regulations

Compliance with labeling regulations is crucial for legal marketing and customer safety. Begin by familiarizing yourself with the regulations that apply to cosmetic products in your region. For example, the U.S. Food and Drug Administration (FDA) has specific requirements for ingredient listing, claims, and packaging for cosmetics.

Ensure that your label includes all mandatory information, such as the product name, net quantity, and manufacturer details. Ingredient lists should be accurate and follow the International Nomenclature of Cosmetic Ingredients (INCI) system. This ensures consistency and clarity in ingredient labeling across different products and brands.

Stay updated with any changes in regulatory requirements to maintain compliance. Regularly review guidelines from relevant authorities and make necessary adjustments to your labeling practices. Non-compliance can result in fines or product recalls, so it's essential to prioritize accurate and up-to-date labeling.

Effective branding and marketing strategies can significantly enhance the visibility and appeal of your lip balm. Start by developing a strong brand identity that resonates with your target audience. This includes creating a memorable brand name, logo, and visual style that differentiates your product from competitors.

Leverage social media platforms and online marketing to promote your lip balm. Share engaging content such as behind-the-scenes looks at the production process, customer testimonials, and promotional offers. Collaborate with influencers or bloggers in the beauty and wellness niche to reach a wider audience and build credibility.

Consider offering samples or trial sizes to attract new customers and encourage word-of-mouth referrals. Participate in local markets, trade shows, or beauty events to showcase your product and connect with potential buyers. Utilize attractive and informative packaging to create a positive first impression and reinforce your brand's message.

CHAPTER EIGHT

Storage And Shelf Life Guidelines

Best Practices For Storing Homemade Lip Balm

Storing homemade lip balm correctly is crucial to maintaining its effectiveness and safety. Begin by ensuring that your lip balm containers are thoroughly clean and dry before filling them. Any moisture or residue can cause the balm to spoil prematurely. Opt for small, airtight containers to prevent exposure to air, which can lead to oxidation and a decrease in quality. Glass or high-quality plastic containers with tight-fitting lids are ideal for this purpose.

Store your lip balm in a cool, dry place away from direct sunlight and heat sources. High temperatures can cause the lip balm to melt or separate, while sunlight can degrade the natural ingredients, reducing their efficacy. A pantry or cupboard is often a suitable location. For those living in warmer climates, consider refrigerating the lip balm to maintain its consistency and extend its shelf life.

It's also beneficial to label your lip balm containers with the date of production. This practice helps you keep track of how long the balm has been stored and ensures you use it within a reasonable timeframe. This simple step can help you manage your lip balm inventory and avoid using products that may no longer be at their best.

Understanding Shelf Life And Expiration Dates

The shelf life of homemade lip balm varies depending on the ingredients used and the storage conditions.

Generally, lip balms made with natural ingredients and without preservatives have a shelf life of about 6 to 12 months. However, if you include preservatives or essential oils known for their longevity, such as vitamin E, you might extend this period slightly. It's important to understand that shelf life refers to the time during which the lip balm remains effective and safe to use, not the point at which it becomes harmful.

Expiration dates are not always straightforward for homemade products. Unlike commercial products with standardized testing and labeling, homemade lip balms rely on ingredient quality and storage practices. Observe the lip balm for any changes in color, texture, or smell, as these are indicators of potential spoilage. If the lip balm has an off odor or shows signs of mold, it's best to discard it.

Regularly check the lip balm for any changes in its consistency or appearance. Solidification, separation, or a grainy texture could signal that the product is past its prime. To ensure you use the balm while it's still effective, keep track of the date you made it and aim to use it within the recommended timeframe.

Tips For Extending Shelf Life

Extending the shelf life of your homemade lip balm can be achieved through several methods. Firstly, incorporating natural preservatives like vitamin E or rosemary extract can help combat the effects of oxidation and microbial growth. These additives not only help preserve the balm but also add beneficial properties to your lips.

Secondly, ensure that your lip balm is kept in optimal condition. Avoid touching the balm with dirty hands or applying it directly from the container if you have a cold sore or other infections, as this can introduce bacteria. Using a small applicator or spatula can help maintain hygiene and prevent contamination.

Finally, consider the type of oils and butter used in your lip balm. Some oils have a longer shelf life than others. For instance, jojoba oil and coconut oil have natural preservative qualities that can contribute to a longer-lasting balm. When selecting ingredients, choose those known for their stability and longevity to maximize the shelf life of your product.

Testing Your Lip Balm For Freshness

Testing your lip balm for freshness involves both sensory evaluation and practical application. Start by inspecting the balm visually. Look for any discoloration, separation, or unusual texture changes that might indicate spoilage.

A well-preserved lip balm should have a uniform appearance without any visible mold or discoloration.

Next, smell the lip balm. Fresh lip balm should have a pleasant, mild scent corresponding to its ingredients. If you detect any sour, rancid, or otherwise unpleasant odors, this is a clear sign that the lip balm may have gone bad. Trust your nose; if it smells off, it's best to err on the side of caution and discard it.

Finally, apply a small amount of the lip balm to your lips or wrist. Fresh lip balm should glide on smoothly and feel moisturizing. If you notice any graininess, separation, or a sticky, unpleasant texture, it might be time to throw it out. Regularly testing your lip balm helps ensure you are only using products that are safe and effective.

Knowing when to discard old batches of lip balm is key to maintaining product quality and safety. As a general rule, if your lip balm has been stored for longer than 12 months or shows any signs of spoilage, it's time to dispose of it. This includes changes in color, texture, or odor, as well as any visible mold or separation.

If you observe that the lip balm no longer performs as expected—such as becoming less effective at moisturizing or showing signs of uneven application—it may also be time to discard it. Even if the balm looks and smells fine, changes in performance can indicate that it has lost its beneficial properties.

Finally, if you have a batch of lip balm that you can't recall making within the past year, it's safer to discard it.

Regularly rotating your stock and keeping accurate records of production dates can help manage your lip balm inventory effectively and avoid using outdated products.

CHAPTER NINE

Using And Enjoying Your Homemade Lip Balm

Applying Lip Balm For Maximum Effectiveness

When applying homemade lip balm, start by ensuring your lips are clean and dry. Any residual food, drink, or lip products can hinder the balm's effectiveness. Gently exfoliate your lips if they are dry or flaky, using a soft toothbrush or a lip scrub. This will help remove dead skin cells and ensure the lip balm adheres better.

Apply a small amount of lip balm to your lips using your fingertip or an applicator if you prefer. Smooth it evenly over your lips, covering the entire surface.

For best results, apply the balm in a thin, even layer. Avoid applying too much, as this can lead to a greasy feeling rather than a smooth finish. Reapply as needed throughout the day, especially after eating or drinking, to maintain hydration and protection.

For those who have sensitive lips or are prone to chapped lips, consider applying a thicker layer of balm before bed. This will provide a more substantial barrier against overnight dryness and help your lips recover more effectively. If you're using your balm for the first time, test it on a small area to ensure there are no adverse reactions.

Benefits Of Using Natural Ingredients

Natural ingredients in lip balm offer several benefits over synthetic alternatives. Ingredients like beeswax, shea butter, and coconut oil are known for their nourishing and moisturizing properties. Beeswax provides a protective barrier that helps lock in moisture, while shea butter and coconut oil deeply hydrates and soothes the lips.

By using natural ingredients, you avoid potentially harmful chemicals and artificial additives found in commercial lip balms. This can be particularly beneficial for those with sensitive skin or allergies. Additionally, natural lip balms often contain antioxidants and vitamins that can promote healthier skin and prevent premature aging.

Natural ingredients are also more environmentally friendly. Many commercially produced lip balms use synthetic ingredients and packaging that contribute to environmental pollution. By choosing natural ingredients and eco-friendly packaging, you contribute to a more sustainable and responsible beauty routine.

Incorporating Lip Balm Into Your Skincare Routine

Integrating your homemade lip balm into your skincare routine is simple and effective. Begin by applying it as part of your morning routine to protect your lips from daily environmental factors such as wind and sun exposure. This ensures your lips are hydrated and ready to face the day.

Consider using the lip balm before applying lipstick or gloss. This creates a smooth base, preventing your lipstick from settling into fine lines and improving its overall appearance. Additionally, you can apply the balm before bed to keep your lips hydrated overnight.

For those who use other skincare products, such as facial moisturizers or sunscreens, ensure the lip balm complements these products. If your skincare routine involves exfoliating or using acids, apply the lip balm after these steps to lock in moisture and protect your lips from potential irritation.

Sharing Your Creations With Friends And Family

Sharing your homemade lip balm with friends and family can be a delightful and personal gesture. Consider packaging your lip balm in small, attractive containers or tins. You can personalize these containers with labels or decorations to make them even more special.

When gifting your lip balm, include a note detailing the natural ingredients used and their benefits. This information adds a personal touch and helps recipients appreciate the effort and care put into the creation. You might also provide tips on how to use the lip balm effectively and how to incorporate it into their skincare routines.

Organize a DIY lip balm party where friends and family can create their lip balms with your guidance. This not only makes for a fun and engaging activity but also allows everyone to learn more about the process and the benefits of natural skincare.

Feedback And Tips From Experienced Users

Listening to feedback from experienced users can provide valuable insights into perfecting your homemade lip balm. Many users recommend experimenting with different natural ingredients to find the ideal combination for their skin type and preferences. For instance, adding essential oils can enhance the balm's scent and offer additional therapeutic benefits.

Experienced users often suggest maintaining consistency in the formulation to ensure the best results. Keeping notes on your ingredient ratios and any adjustments made will help you refine your recipe over time. Additionally, pay attention to any changes in texture or scent, as these can indicate that a component needs adjustment.

Consider joining online forums or local groups dedicated to DIY beauty products. These communities are great resources for sharing experiences, receiving tips, and staying updated on the latest trends and techniques. Engaging with other enthusiasts can also inspire new ideas and improvements for your homemade lip balm.

CHAPTER TEN

Advanced Lip Balm Techniques And Recipes

Formulating Specialty Lip Balms

Creating specialty lip balms requires a thoughtful approach to ingredient selection and formulation. For healing lip balms, you'll want to include ingredients known for their restorative properties. For instance, calendula and chamomile extracts are renowned for their soothing and healing effects on the skin. You can infuse these extracts into your base oils by gently heating them with a double boiler. Similarly, adding essential oils like tea tree or lavender can enhance the balm's therapeutic properties.

Plumping lip balms often incorporate ingredients that stimulate circulation and provide a fuller appearance. Consider using peppermint or cinnamon essential oils, which can create a tingling sensation that may temporarily plump the lips. Ensure these oils are used in moderation, as they can be quite potent. Combine these essential oils with hydrating components like hyaluronic acid to maintain moisture and give your lips a fuller look.

To formulate these balms, start by melting your base (such as beeswax or candelilla wax) with a carrier oil like coconut or jojoba oil. Once melted, add your specialty ingredients and stir thoroughly. Pour the mixture into lip balm tubes or containers and let it cool completely before use. This process ensures that the active ingredients are well-integrated into the balm and provide the desired effects.

Advanced lip balm recipes often incorporate exotic oils and butter to create luxurious and effective products. Oils such as argan, marula, and rosehip are not only rich in nutrients but also offer unique benefits for lip care. Argan oil, for instance, is high in Vitamin E and essential fatty acids, making it excellent for moisturizing and repairing lips. Marula oil, known for its high antioxidant content, can help protect lips from environmental damage.

When using these oils, start by substituting them for more common carrier oils in your base recipe. For instance, replace sweet almond oil with argan oil or blend it with other exotic oils for a unique combination. Butter like mango or shea butter can also be used to enhance the balm's texture and provide additional moisturizing benefits.

This butter can be melted along with your wax and carrier oils to create a smooth, creamy balm.

To incorporate these ingredients effectively, consider creating a small test batch first. This allows you to experiment with ratios and ensure that the exotic oils blend well with your base. Keep track of the proportions used and any observations about texture or scent. Once satisfied with your formulation, scale up to produce larger batches for personal use or sharing.

Creating Themed Collections

Creating themed collections adds a fun and creative touch to your lip balm offerings. Seasonal flavors, such as pumpkin spice for fall or peppermint mocha for winter, can be achieved by infusing your base with specific flavoring agents and essential oils.

For example, to create a pumpkin spice lip balm, use pumpkin seed oil for its rich texture and combine it with spices like cinnamon, nutmeg, and clove, carefully measuring to avoid overpowering flavors.

For a summer collection, consider fruity flavors like watermelon or tropical coconut. Use natural flavor oils or extracts to achieve these flavors without adding artificial ingredients. Experiment with blending these flavors in small batches to find the perfect balance. You can also add colorants derived from natural sources, such as beet juice or spirulina powder, to give your lip balms a vibrant appearance.

Themed collections can be presented in attractive packaging that reflects the season or theme. Create custom labels and use decorative containers to enhance the appeal. This approach not only makes your lip balms more engaging but also provides an excellent opportunity for gifts or special promotions.

Developing Personalized Lip Balm Recipes

Personalizing lip balm recipes involves tailoring them to specific preferences or needs. Start by identifying what you want in your custom balm—whether it's a unique flavor, color, or specific skin benefits. For instance, if you have sensitive skin, you might opt for a balm with soothing ingredients like chamomile and unscented base oils to minimize irritation.

Begin by experimenting with different base recipes and adjust the ratios of wax, oils, and butter to suit your preferences. Test various essential oils for fragrance and therapeutic benefits, keeping in mind that some may be more suitable for sensitive skin than others.

Record your experiments meticulously, noting the ingredient amounts and any adjustments made.

Once you have a preferred recipe, consider creating a batch and conducting a patch test to ensure it meets your expectations. This process allows you to refine the recipe further if needed. Developing personalized recipes can be a rewarding experience as it enables you to create a lip balm that perfectly suits your needs or the needs of a loved one.

Tips For Starting A Small Lip Balm Business

Starting a small lip balm business involves more than just creating great products—it also requires planning and strategy. Begin by researching your target market and identifying a niche. Are you focusing on organic ingredients, luxury formulations, or unique flavors?

Understanding your audience will help tailor your products and marketing efforts.

Develop a business plan outlining your production process, sourcing of ingredients, and packaging options. Consider the costs involved, including raw materials, equipment, and labeling. Ensuring your products comply with local regulations and obtaining necessary certifications can also be crucial for selling your lip balms commercially.

Marketing your lip balm business effectively involves creating a strong brand presence. Utilize social media platforms to showcase your products, share customer reviews, and engage with potential buyers. Offering promotions or samples can help attract initial customers and build a loyal client base. As your business grows, consider expanding your product line or exploring new distribution channels to reach a broader audience.

By following these steps and maintaining a focus on quality and customer satisfaction, you can successfully launch and grow a small lip balm business.

In conclusion, the exploration of lip balm reveals its importance as a multifaceted product that goes beyond mere cosmetic appeal. Its primary function is to protect and nourish the lips, making it an essential part of personal care routines. Whether addressing the needs of individuals with dry, chapped lips or those seeking to maintain lip health, lip balm provides a crucial barrier against environmental factors such as wind, sun, and extreme temperatures.

The formulation of lip balm has evolved significantly over the years, with advancements in ingredients and technology enhancing its effectiveness. Modern lip balms are crafted with a variety of ingredients, including natural oils, waxes, and butter, which offer a range of benefits from hydration to long-lasting moisture. Ingredients like beeswax, shea butter, and coconut oil not only moisturize but also create a protective layer that helps retain moisture, ensuring that lips stay soft and supple.

Moreover, lip balms often incorporate additional features such as SPF protection, which is crucial for shielding the lips from harmful UV rays. This added benefit underscores the product's role in comprehensive lip care, addressing both immediate and long-term health needs. Some formulations also include therapeutic agents like menthol or camphor, which can provide soothing relief for irritated lips, highlighting the versatility of lip balms in catering to various conditions.

The market for lip balms is diverse, reflecting the wide range of preferences and needs among consumers. From tinted balms that add a hint of color to those with medicinal properties for treating specific issues, the variety ensures that there is a suitable option for everyone. Additionally, the rise of eco-friendly and sustainable packaging options represents a growing awareness of environmental impact, aligning with broader consumer trends towards sustainability.

In essence, lip balm is more than a simple cosmetic product; it is a practical tool for maintaining lip health and comfort. Its development has mirrored advances in skincare, emphasizing the importance of high-quality ingredients and thoughtful formulation. As consumer preferences continue to evolve, the future of lip balm will likely see further innovations, enhancing its functionality and appeal.

Ultimately, incorporating lip balm into daily routines can significantly contribute to overall lip care, offering protection, hydration, and comfort.

Its role in personal grooming and wellness underscores its value, making it a staple in many individuals' personal care arsenals.

THE END